Anke Rüsbüldt

Vaccination and Worming of Horses

What you need to know

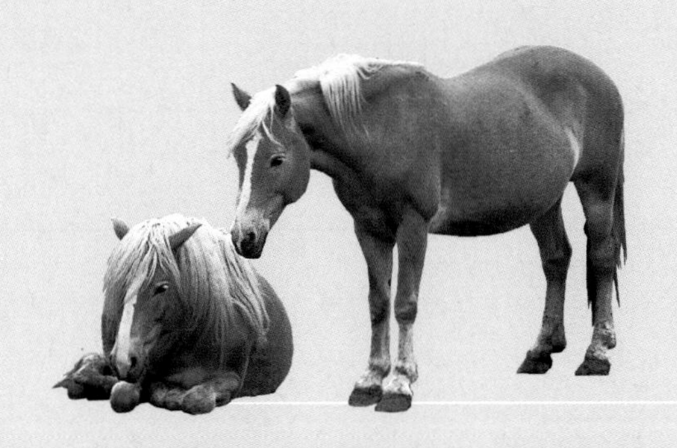

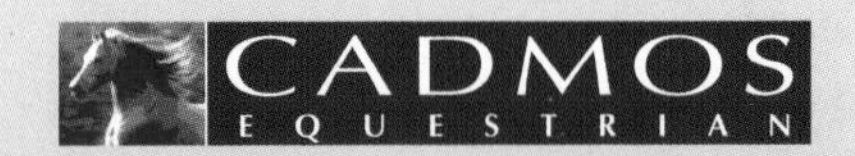

Contents

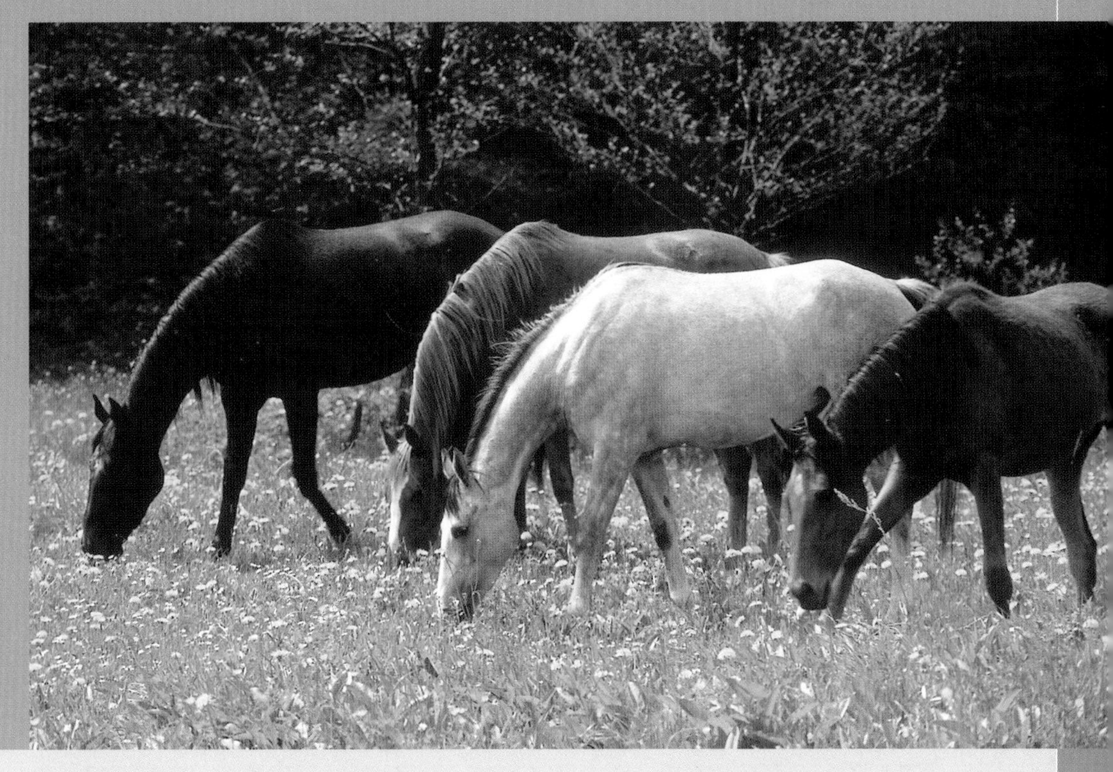

Grazing in a herd can lead to infection.
Photo: C. Koller

Keeping a Healthy Horse

Keeping horses is a major responsibility. Caring for them properly includes everything from providing proper feed and stabling, together with appropriate exercise, to looking after their health. To say "My horse is healthy, he hasn't needed to see a vet in years" is not only an indication of poor management, but also demonstrates a failure to take seriously an owner's responsibilities in keeping a horse.

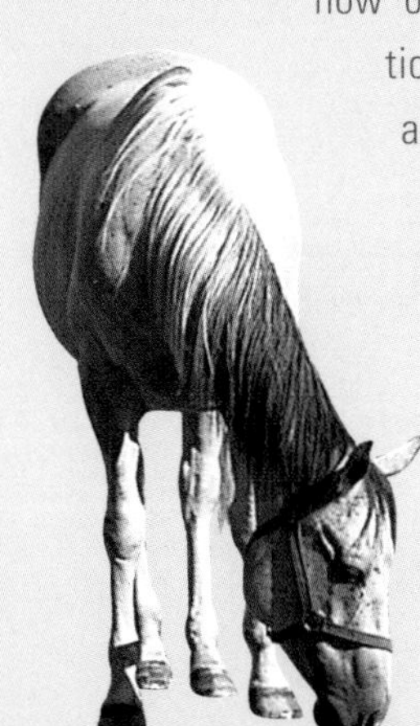

Apart from normal care and hygiene, routine precautions to safeguard your horse's health should include daily observation, an annual health check (including teeth), and regular vaccination and worming. Why horses should be vaccinated and wormed, how often, and against which infections, is what this guide is all about. Because of the way we keep them, horses are highly susceptible to infection. Given that we are directly responsible for the care of our horses, it follows that we should give them every opportunity to avoid infection.

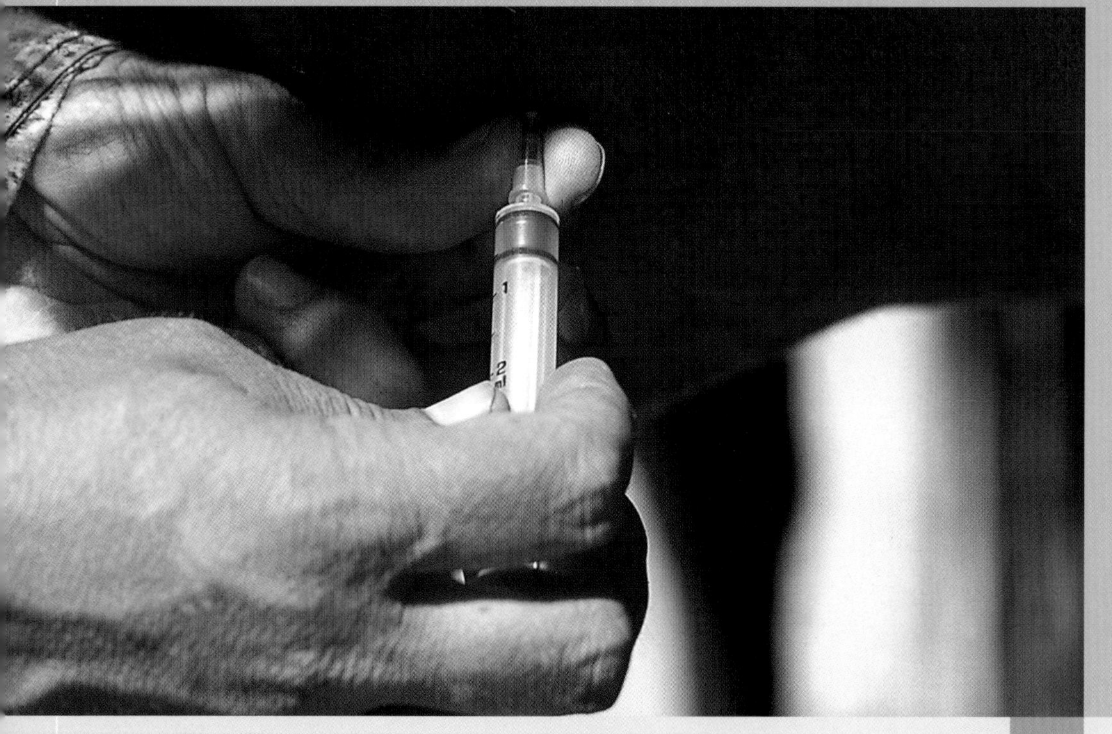

Regular vaccination can protect against illness .
Photo: S. Stuewer

Infectious Illnesses

There are a number of infectious illnesses that a horse owner can have his horse vaccinated against. These include tetanus, equine flu, herpes, rabies and fungal skin infections.

Tip

For optimal protection, it is a good idea to have all horses in the stable vaccinated against the same illnesses.

Tetanus

Every horse should be vaccinated against tetanus. The chances of a horse contracting the disease are slim, but the risks associated with this happening are just too great to ignore. Horses are far more susceptible to tetanus than many other animals. The tetanus bacterium, *clostridium tetani*, is found everywhere – in the paddock, in bedding, in arenas, and on stable floors.

Horses can become infected with tetanus through any wound. This need not be a large or gaping wound, a small scrape is enough. Coronet injuries, wounds made by nails or wire, and small scrapes picked up in the paddock which we rarely even notice, are perfect pathways for tetanus. The tetanus bacterium thrives in anaerobic conditions where there is no oxygen.

When a horse becomes infected with tetanus, death is almost inevitable. In a few cases the horse will survive, but as a rule, infection is followed by death, and the horse dies suffering. Writers and other who claim that horses can develop a natural immunity are simply wrong. Anyone unlucky enough to see a horse die from tetanus will always insist on vaccination.

Vaccination programme: Primary vaccinations should be given starting at five months of age, twice within 4–8 weeks, the third time at the age of one year old, and thereafter once every 24 months.

If a horse is injured and no one knows whether it has been vaccinated or not, both the tetanus vaccine and tetanus serum should be given, to be on the safe side. This is also the case where horses of uncertain vaccination status are to be castrated. However, this alone cannot guarantee protection and the horses should be given primary immunisations where possible.

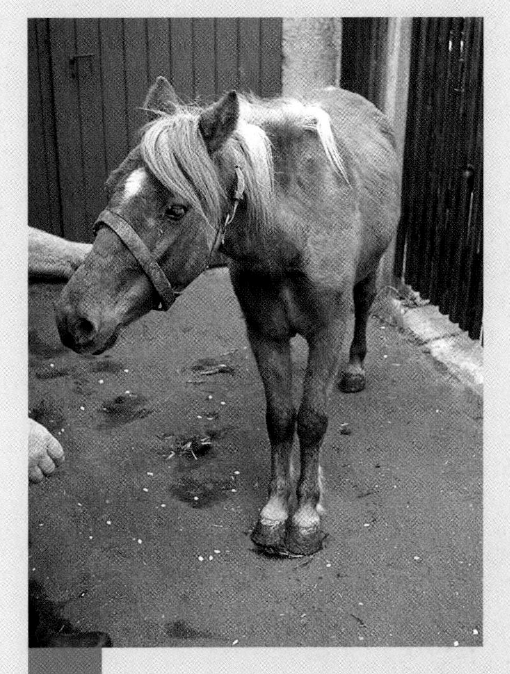

This pony has a tetanus infection: vaccination could have saved it from this deadly illness. Photo: H. Ende

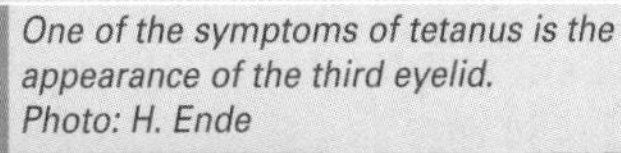

One of the symptoms of tetanus is the appearance of the third eyelid. Photo: H. Ende

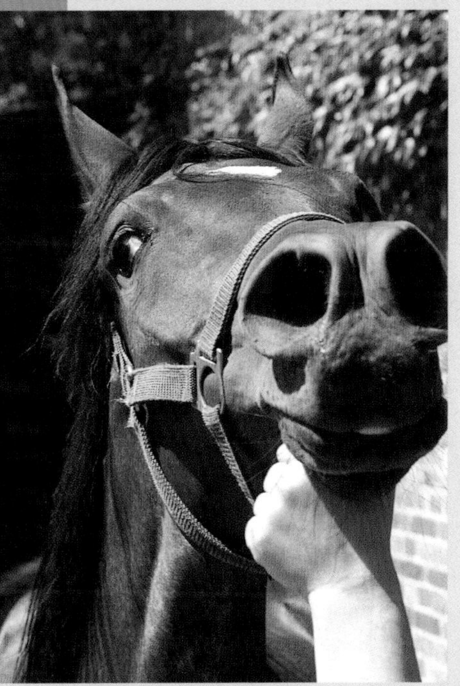

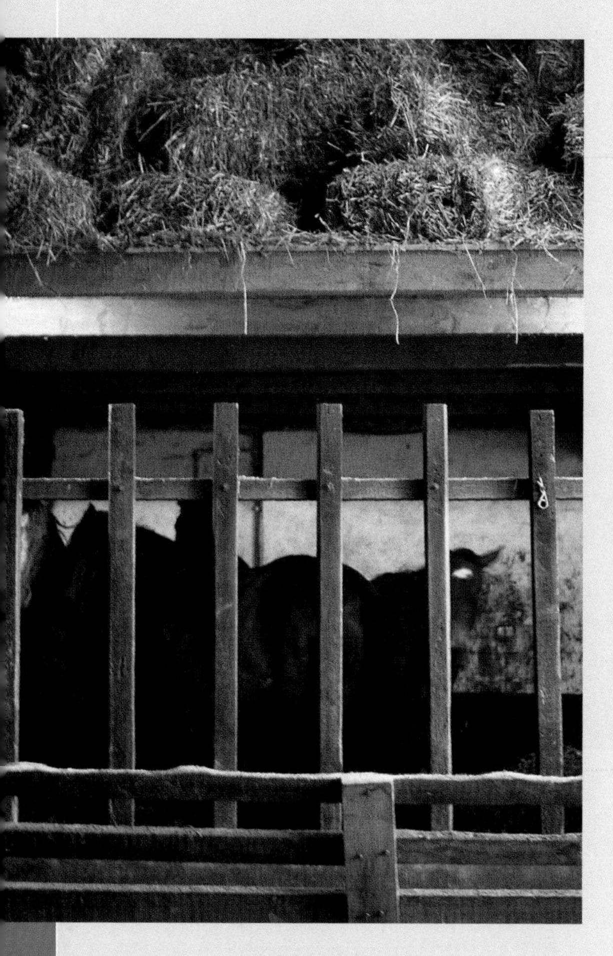

These conditions are less than ideal: the dust from the hay puts undue strain on the airways of the horses. Photo: H. Ende

Mouldy hay is harmful to the airways, and can lead to colic. Photo: H. Ende

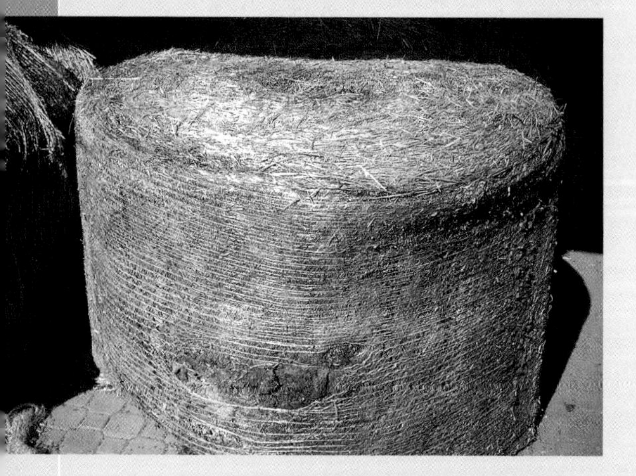

Tip

These days, no horse need die from tetanus

Combined vaccinations are available against both tetanus and equine flu. This type of vaccination is often used after the primary immunisation has been done. The combination vaccine can be used every two years, and in between horses should be given the single vaccination against flu (see below). Too many tetanus shots can be detrimental to a horse's health.

Influenza

Influenza, also known as epidemic cough, equine flu and Newmarket cough, is an acute viral infection of the airways. It is caused by one of a variety of orthomyxoviruses which multiply in the mucous membranes of infected animals and are transmitted through the air. It is characterised by coughing and high fever, and spreads almost epidemically. The virus has two subtypes – the first type stays relatively constant, and the other changes in response to various mechanisms. New variants can suddenly appear and cause a new epidemic. For this reason, the vaccine has to be constantly modified, improved and adapted to suit the current infections.

All vaccines available on the market contain inactivated viruses or parts of viruses. No live vaccines are used for influenza. Some

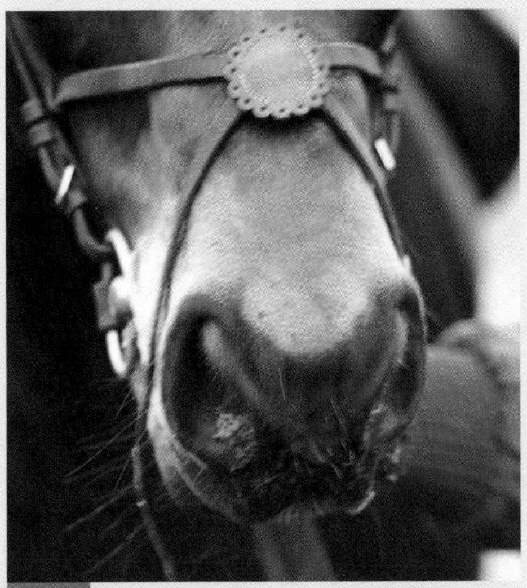

*Nosebleed is often a sign of concealed airway illnesses.
Photo: H. Ende*

vaccines contain so-called immune stimulating complexes (ISCOMs). These boost the immune system by encouraging the development of additional defence cells. In order for a vaccine to give the best level of protection, it must include a number of relevant viruses. There are types 1 and 2, and a whole range of subtypes, which are named after their places of origin. The labelling reflects the complexity of vaccines, for example: "inactivated antigens for Influenza virus A/Equi 1/Prague/1/56, A/Equi 2/Miami/63, A/Equi 2/Newmarket/2/93".

These vaccines can only function effectively when the primary vaccination has been carried out correctly and the regular boosters have been kept up to date.

Remember that these vaccinations on the one hand protect your own horse against the illness, and on the other help to prevent the epidemic spread of influenza amongst the wider horse population. The more horses that are vaccinated, the better. From an epidemiological point of view, it is preferable for all horses to be vaccinated.

Of course, you hear opinions from holistic doctors in human medicine, and practitioners of natural medicine and alternative therapies, who are against vaccination. They are entitled to their opinions. Should you decide, as an individual horse owner, not to vaccinate you ought to consider, besides the infection possibilities, what would happen if everyone did that. If your unvaccinated horse does escape becoming infected, it could well be that the disease simply never reached your stables because all the other horses in your area were already vaccinated.

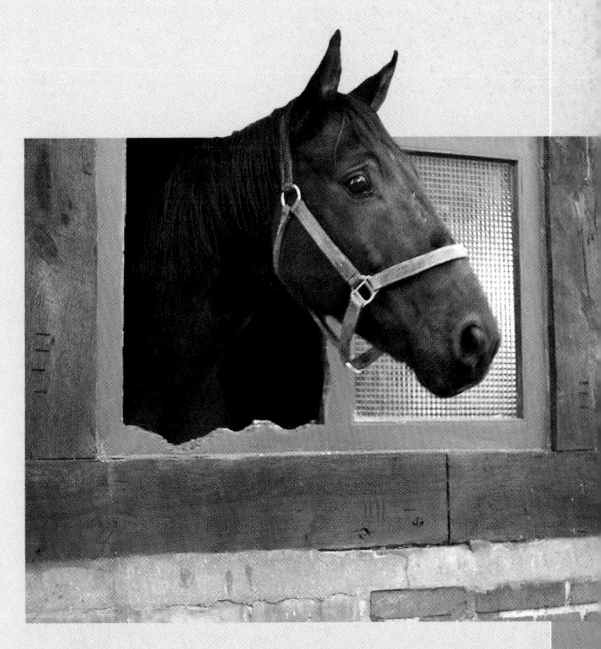

Fresh air is ideal, although this window poses the danger of injury. Photo: H. Ende

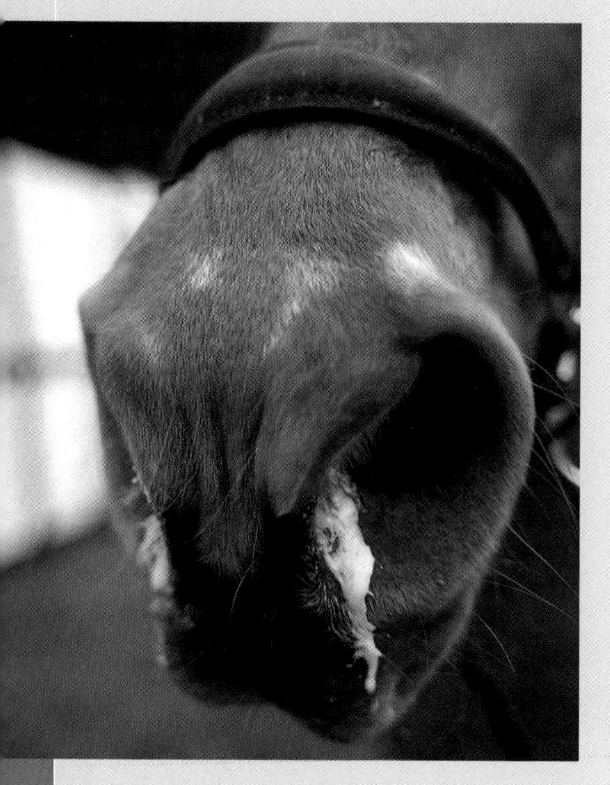

White discharge from the nostrils should be investigated. Photo: H. Ende

Of course, you hear opinions from holistic doctors in human medicine, and practitioners of natural medicine and alternative therapies, who are against vaccination. They are entitled to their opinions. Should you decide, as an individual horse owner, not to vaccinate you ought to consider, besides the infection possibilities, what would happen if everyone did that. If your unvaccinated horse does escape becoming infected, it could well be that the disease simply never reached your stables because all the other horses in your area were already vaccinated.

If you take steps to boost your horse's immune system both before and during vaccination, you can help your horse to cope better

Tip

Give your horse three days of rest after vaccination.

with vaccination. Ways to help includes giving your horse three full days of rest after vaccination, and postponing the vaccination if the horse is under any kind of stress. For example, try not to vaccinate your horse the day after a show, as even experienced competition horses get stressed at shows, and the stress takes a few days to dissipate. Another consideration to take into account is that all the other horses at shows carry numerous bacteria with them, which means that your own horse's immune system is already being tested to the limit.

Your horse should, at the time of vaccination, be healthy and free of parasites (e.g. worms). It is recommended that you have your horse checked and wormed before vaccination, rather than the other way round.

If you are a competitor at shows or events, the organisers will often ask to see the horse's vaccination certificate. In most cases, it will only be accepted if the horse has had its primary vaccinations and its regular boosters. Most livery stables and pony clubs will therefore also have regular vaccination programmes.

Foals of vaccinated mares receive adequate protection from their mother's antibodies, which lasts up to their fifth month. Vaccination should be given when the foals have only a few maternal antibodies left. The second vaccination is given four to six weeks after the first one and the third vaccination four to six months thereafter. A booster vaccination should be given every six to twelve months, according to the manufacturer's instructions. Most manufacturers note that the effective duration of vaccination significantly shortens in stressful situations (such as at shows). As a result, some organisations expect competitors to maintain vaccinations at roughly six monthly intervals.

Combination vaccinations are available on the market for influenza and tetanus, or influenza and herpes.

Equine herpes

Herpes infections are implicated in abortion, delivery of stillborn foals, venereal infections and eye disease. Next to influenza, the herpes virus is the most common viral disease in horses. Most of the horse population in mainland Europe has already been exposed to the herpes virus. Apart from the serious and acute illnesses it causes, there are also latent and chronic infections. In stress situations, or when other horses become ill, the latent infection can be become an acute infection.

Tip

Modern vaccines are well tolerated by healthy horses. There need be no undue concern about side effects arising from vaccination.

There are different types of equine herpes. The main viruses are EHV1 and EHV4. EHV1 causes epidemic abortions, neurological problems and airway illnesses. EHV4 mainly causes illnesses of the upper airways. The two viruses are quite similar and show some cross-immunity. There are live vaccines for EHV1, and inactive vaccines for EHV1 and EHV4. Combined vaccines mostly contain inactive EHV1 and EHV4 as well as some influenza strains.

With both primary immunisation and boosters, it is important to always study the label or data sheet, as incorrect vaccination can be as bad as no vaccination.

The protection of each horse can only be guaranteed when a vaccination programme is carried out regularly as prescribed, and all animals are included. Some show organisations demand herpes vaccinations as a rule, especially if there are breeding programmes on the property.

Vaccination programme: Primary immunisation starts in the third month. Repeat combination vaccination after four to eight weeks, then again after four to six months. Thereafter boosters are given every six to eight months. EHV1 live vaccination should be repeated after three months, and thereafter every six to nine months.

Pregnant mares should be vaccinated in the third

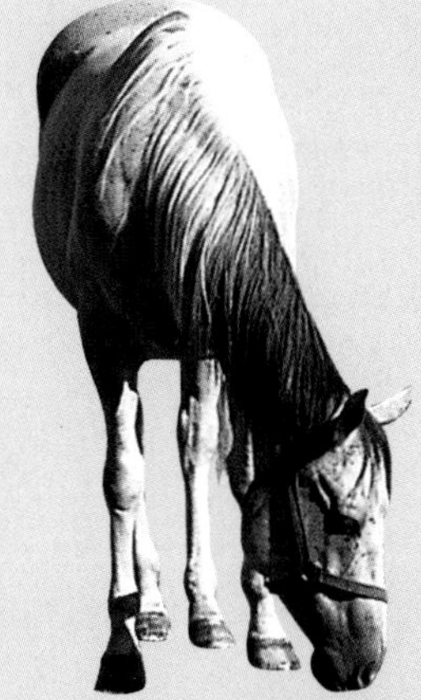

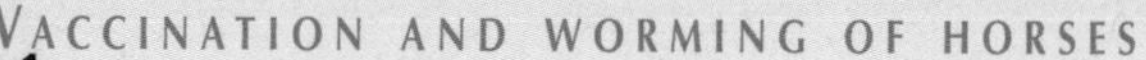

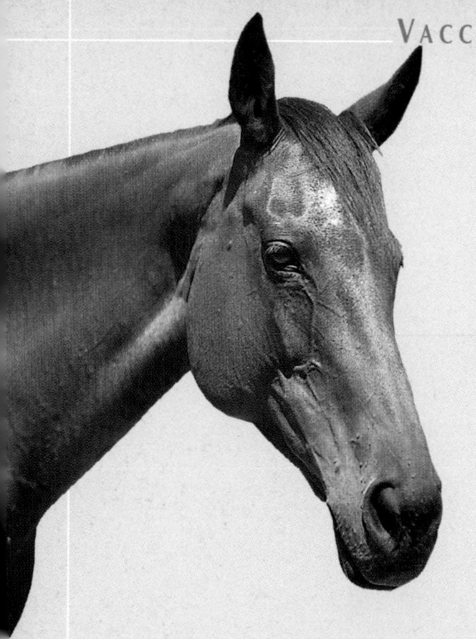

or fourth month of pregnancy, and again at seven to nine months (but always read the manufacturer's instructions and also the rules of any associations of which you are a member). A change of vaccination or delay in administration can alter the protection given by the vaccination.

As with influenza vaccination, owners of single horses which are always kept far enough away from other horses can opt to avoid vaccination completely.

Only healthy horses should be vaccinated: not horses with parasitic infestations or under any stress. Three days' rest is suggested. This does not have to mean three days in the stable, but three days' rest from work that makes them sweat, so gentle hacking may be allowed.

Tip

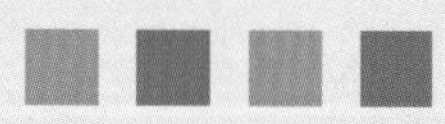

All vaccinations are recorded on a vaccination certificate. See that this is available at all times, preferably close to where your horse is stabled.

Rabies

In regions where rabies is endemic, your horse should be vaccinated. This does not apply in the United Kingdom, but if you plan to travel overseas with your horse, consult your vet or agricultural organisation for information. Rabies in horses is rare but always deadly. The disease is extremely dangerous to humans and attempted treatment of sick animals is prohibited. Cases of rabies must be reported to the authorities.

Vaccination programme: Vaccination is to be done once a year starting from the age of six months.

Fungal skin infections

It is only recently that a vaccination against fungal skin infections in domestic animals has appeared on the market. Unusually, this vaccination may also be effective in horses already suffering from a fungal disease. The range of problems this vaccination is effective for is a matter of some controversy at the moment, but it has been said that it can help against summer sores, diarrhoea and allergic coughs. Whether this is in fact so has not yet been adequately researched.

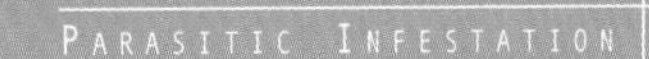

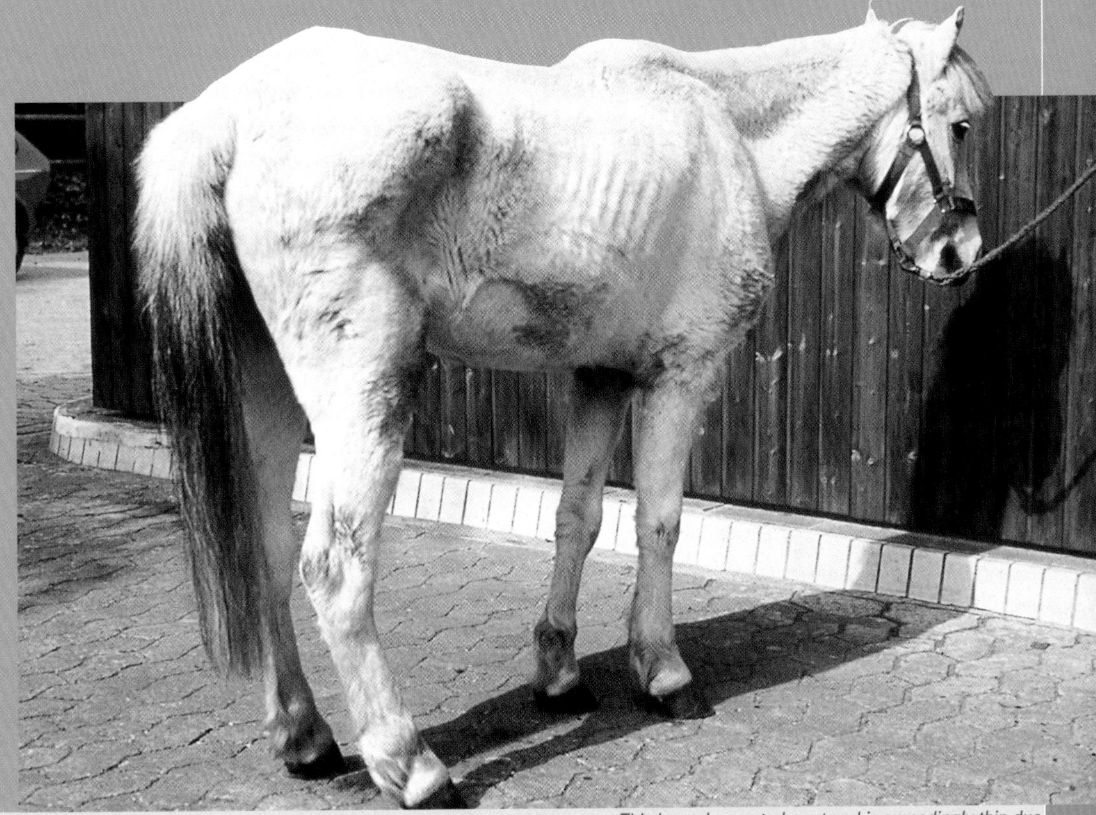

This horse has a stark coat and is exceedingly thin due to worm infestation. It should never get this far.
Photo: H. Ende

Vaccination programme: Vaccination is done twice in a fortnight. You should be aware that with the second vaccination, there is the possibility of fever and swelling. Protection lasts for about one year.

Parasitic Infestations

Worm infestation has always been a problem in horses, and a regular worming regime is standard practice for most horse owners. In spite of this, the worm problem is difficult to control.

Keeping horses in herds, in pastures that are used too frequently and too intensively, provides an ideal environment for worm

Tip

As a rule, worm infestation remains hidden. By the time you see worms in the droppings, or weight loss and diarrhoea are noticed, it is often too late. Please do not allow it to progress that far.

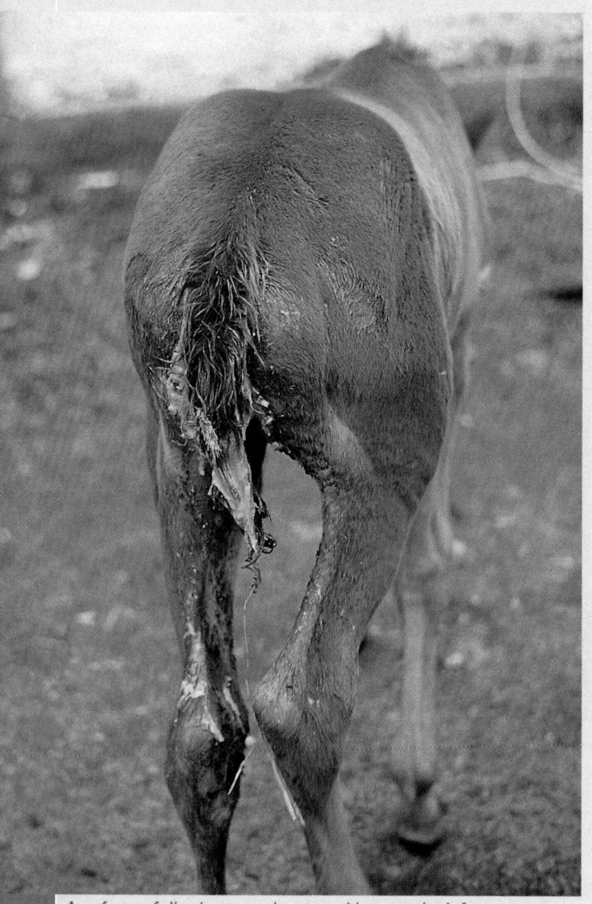
Any form of diarrhoea can be caused by parasite infestation. Ultimately, it can be deadly.
Photo: H. Ende

This horse is critically ill due to acute parasite infestation. Photo: H. Ende

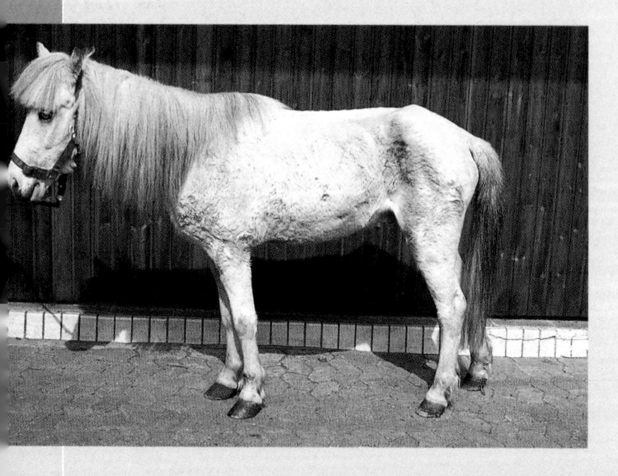

Tip

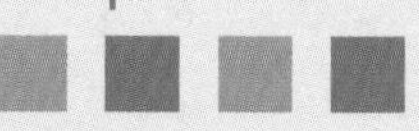

Symptoms attributed to intolerance to medication can in reality often be blamed on worms in the intestines. When following a sensible worming programme, such reactions rarely occur.

infestations. The other problems are the resistance that worms develop to preventative medication, plus poor hygiene and inadequate worming strategies. Deadly illnesses can be caused by worms, with significant parasitic infestation implicated in more than half of all cases of colic, even in horses that are regularly wormed. Tests have shown that there are almost invariably a considerable number of parasites present.

It is important to develop a broad knowledge of worms and their life cycles, and to have an effective worming strategy. The worming plan should include all the horses that share the same pastures. The medication that is available nowadays has been extensively tes-ted and is very well tolerated. The myth that too much worming poses a risk to horses is dangerous: having too many worms is much more hazardous.

Homoeopathic or "natural" cures unfortunately tend not to be very successful. The idea that a horse can be kept completely free of parasites is a fallacy. All approaches to parasite control are based on attempting to limit the infestation. A small population of different parasites is always present in any horse, even with the best possible hygiene. It is our responsibility to keep the infestation to a minimum so that it does not harm the health of our horses. Do not be fooled if worms are not visible in the droppings, as most worms are too small to see with the naked eye. The excreted eggs are always too small to be visible, and can only be seen when examined under a microscope.

Worm parasites

There are many types of worm which can attack, reside in and harm horses. They can be roughly divided into three groups: roundworms (nematodes), tapeworms (cestodes) and insects (bots).

The most numerous and varied of these groups are the roundworms or nematodes. Included in this group are small and large red worms, roundworms, pinworms, threadworms, equine lungworms and hairworms, as well as two types that use insects as intermediate hosts, the stomach worm and filarial nematodes.

Tip

Update your worming programme regularly.

Small red worms (Strongylides)

There are more than 40 different types of strongylides, and they can account for up to 90 per cent of an individual worm infestation. They are 0.5 – 2.5 cm long and are therefore visible to the naked eye. They mostly live in the large intestine and have a relatively simple life cycle. The adult female worm sheds eggs that are deposited in the pasture with the horse's droppings. In the next 5 – 15 days the larvae will develop. The horses ingest these larvae while they graze. The larvae then bore into the wall of the large intestines,

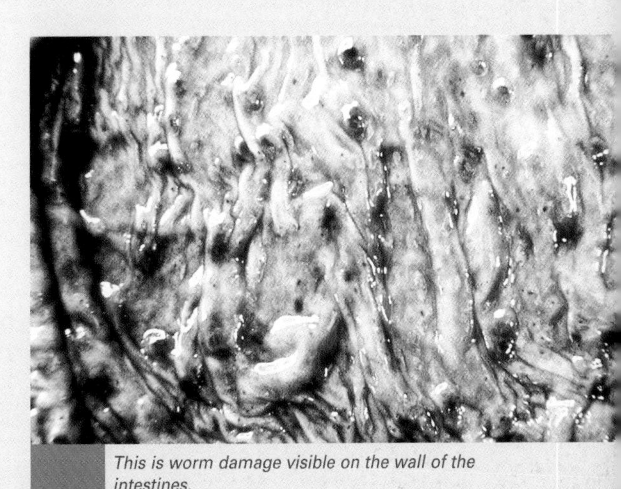

This is worm damage visible on the wall of the intestines.
Photo: Pfitzer GmbH

You cannot see the eggs in the droppings. When you can see worms in the droppings, treatment is urgently needed. Photo: H. Ende

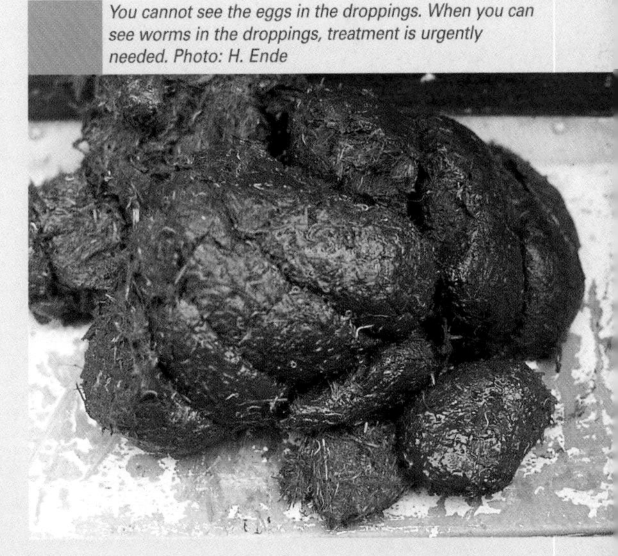

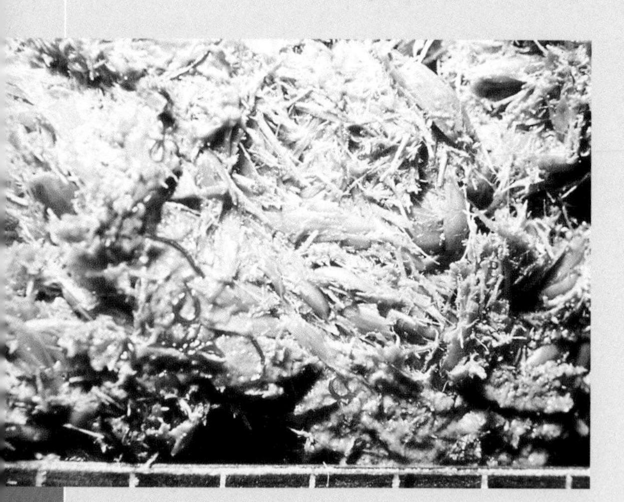

Red worms have established themselves; treatment is essential. Photo: Pfitzer GmbH

re-emerging in about six weeks as mature worms.

It is important to be aware that the small strongylides are typically pasture parasites – these worms do not generally infect horses that are only kept stabled. At one time the practice of mowing pastures was considered advisable, but this did not control the worms because the larvae that were left behind could still make their way to the top of the grass, only to be ingested later. The part of the life cycle during which the larvae are in the walls of the large intestine is also a time when any medication will be ineffective, as these larvae can remain dormant for up to two and a half years in the intestinal walls. Normally there are thousands of larvae hibernating in the intestines during winter, ready to hatch in the spring and cause a serious bout of diarrhoea.

When we actually manage to kill all the adult worms with our worming, we can be sure that new worms will hatch immediately afterwards. This means that we must either use a remedy that is effective in the larvae stage, or repeat the treatment within a short time span.

Some of these worms have the nasty habit of becoming resistant to worming preparations which contain benzimidazole. These drugs will then become ineffective. Serious infestations with small red worms will lead to weight loss, colic, diarrhoea and in extreme cases even death.

Large red worms (Strongylides)

As with the small red worms, there are also many different types of large red worm, of which the most important is the *strongylus vulgaris*, also called the bloodworm. Fortunately this infestation is not as significant a problem as it once was.

The bloodworm is 2.5 cm long. The life cycle starts when eggs, which are shed by the female in the intestines, are deposited with the droppings on the paddock. In the space of two weeks, the eggs develop into larvae that are ingested during grazing. The larvae penetrate the wall of the large intestines and migrate into the small arteries. They then travel against the blood flow until they reach larger arteries. After approximately eleven days, they stop travelling and stick to the walls of the arteries, where they remain for up to four months. After this they migrate, via the bloodstream, back to the intestines and lodge themselves into the intestinal walls for a couple of weeks. When they are settled in the intestines, and if they are not disturbed, they will flourish and produce eggs. Relatives of these worms, also strongylide types, migrate through the liver and pancreas before moving back to the intestines.

These worms cause serious damage during their migration. Damage to the walls of the arteries can lead to thrombosis, causing restriction to the blood flow, spasmodic colic and intermittent lameness. At this stage not much can be done to treat the problem. It is best to try to prevent this situation arising.

Unsurprisingly, the worms also cause damage to the intestines. Intestinal damage causes weight-loss, diarrhoea, loss of appetite and a rough coat. Foals may also get fever and exhaustion, and in severe cases they die.

Roundworms (Ascarids)

The most significant culprit in this group is *parascaris equorum*. These worms can grow to a whopping 20 – 50 cm!

The adult parasites in the intestines shed eggs which are extremely robust. The eggs can survive in the outside world for years, and are only sensitive to high temperatures and certain disinfectants. To top it all, the worms can lay hundreds of thousands of these durable eggs every day. When a horse (or notably a foal) ingests these eggs, the larvae hatch and start to migrate immediately. The first stop is the liver for a week, and then they travel via the bloodstream to the lungs, where they stay for between one and two weeks. After that they emerge from the lungs through the bronchi and airways into the pharynx. They finally migrate back to the intestines via the oesophagus and develop into adult worms. All this takes only 10 – 16 weeks, but the damage done along the way is considerable. The wall of the intestine is damaged, the liver is scarred and parts of the lungs are destroyed. While they are migrating, the larvae are beyond the reach of any medication. Tests on droppings do not necessarily reveal their presence, even when the horse is coughing and has difficulty breathing. The inaccessibility of the larvae and the noteworthy life expectancy of the many eggs mean that roundworm infestation can reinstate itself rapidly. Roundworms can be found everywhere in the horse's environment – they stick to the stable wall, are hidden in the bedding and can even be found on the udders of mares. Foals and young horses are most vulnerable, as their immune systems are not yet at their full strength.

Apart from difficulty in breathing, infested horses can also show the following symp-

Roundworms can cause serious damage. Photo: H. Ende

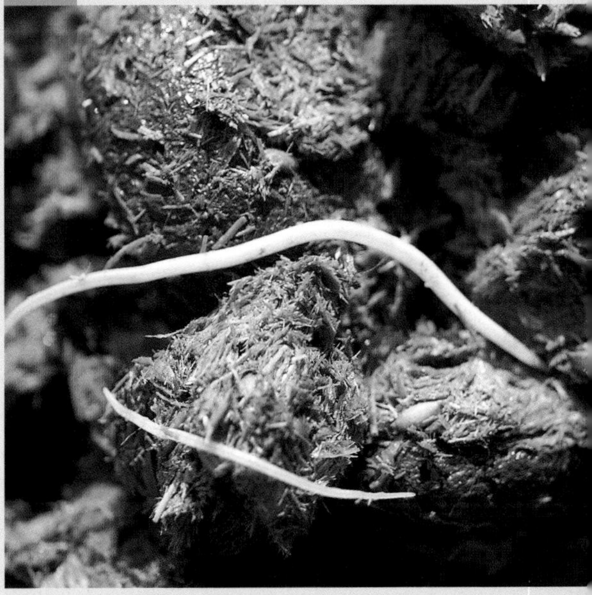

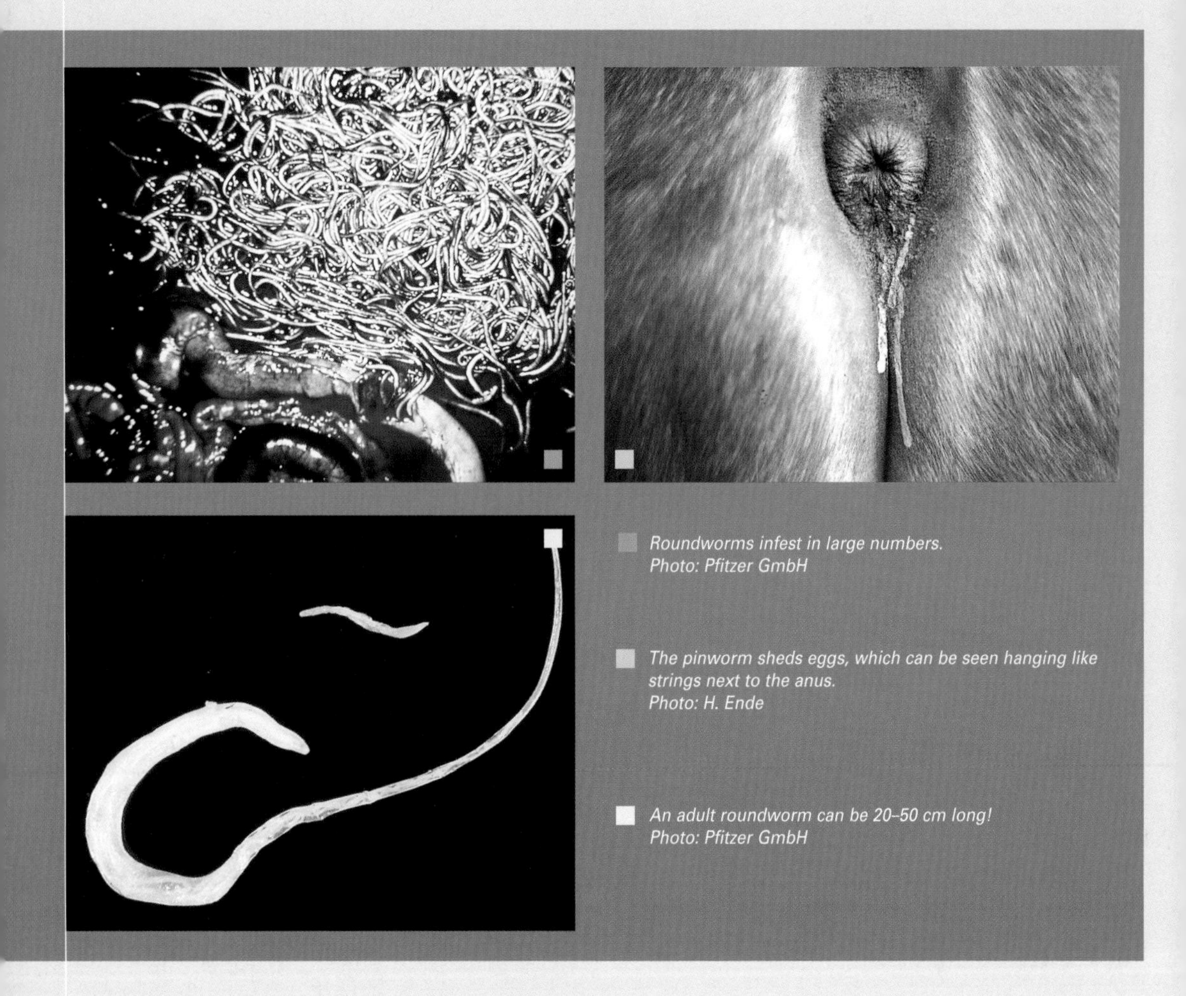

Roundworms infest in large numbers.
Photo: Pfitzer GmbH

The pinworm sheds eggs, which can be seen hanging like strings next to the anus.
Photo: H. Ende

An adult roundworm can be 20–50 cm long!
Photo: Pfitzer GmbH

toms: loss of appetite, apathy, diarrhoea, underdevelopment, dull coat, colic, blockage of the small intestines, and ruptures of the intestines in general.

Pinworms (Oxyuris equi)

Adult pinworms are up to 10 cm long. Their life cycle is approximately four months long and the eggs of these worms can easily be seen. The adult female leaves the gut and sheds stringy-looking eggs next to the rectum. Each stringy egg packet contains up to 50,000 eggs, and adheres to the skin where it can be seen with the naked eye. You can apply some sticky tape to them, pull them off, and give them to your vet to examine under a microscope.

When cleaning the anus, you should always use a separate sponge or, better still, some disposable wipes.

Threadworms (Strongyloides westeri)

These worms are generally harmless in older horses, but can kill foals. With a length of only one cm, the worm's whole life cycle is a mere 8 – 14 days. The danger to newborn foals comes about when the worms are ingested along with the mother's milk, at a time when the foal's immature immune systems is not yet sufficiently active to cope. The result is often diarrhoea, which can end in death. The mild diarrhoea many foals have at two weeks of age is usually not linked to worms, but is more likely related to the mare coming into season again. These worms can also penetrate through the skin of the horse.

In foals, threadworm infestation leads to inflammation of the small intestine, together with diarrhoea and damage to the lungs. Usually, healthy foals will build up a resistance to these worms within the first couple of months of their lives.

Equine lungworms (Dictyocaulus arnfieldi)

The first thing that comes to mind when thinking of lungworm is donkey, which are the favourite host of these worms. They live their whole life cycle of two to eight months in donkeys or foals. The adult worm is up to 8 cm long and can live in the lungs of horses, but cannot reproduce there. It is completely safe to keep donkeys and horses together, as long as both are wormed regularly.

New donkeys being introduced to a herd should be given ivermectin twice in six weeks, and they can then follow the normal worming programme. Take care when calculating dosages relative to weight, as donkeys are relatively light. The normal donkey weighs between 150 and 200 kg (if you own a Poitou, of course, they are heavier).

Hairworms (Trichostrongylus axei)

This worm is very small (0.5 cm) and has a very short life cycle (three weeks). It causes diarrhoea and weight loss. They prefer to use sheep and cattle as hosts, so it will not make any difference to rotate ruminants through the pasture as a preventative measure.

Stomach worms (Habronema muscae)

The adult worm is 3.5 cm long. Larvae that hatch from the eggs are eaten by maggots. The maggots grow into flies, and at the same time the worm larvae reach adulthood. The adult flies deposit the worms on the skin of the horse, where they may be licked off and thus find their way back to the gut again.

Filarial nematodes (Onchocerca cervicalis)

The adult worm is 5 – 30 cm long and lives under the horse's skin. An embryonic larva of the worm, called a microfilaria, is deposited on the horse via a biting fly called *culicoides nubeculosus*. These insects most commonly affect the horse's flanks and spine, causing an itch in these areas when the microfilariae are living under the skin. Microfilariae can

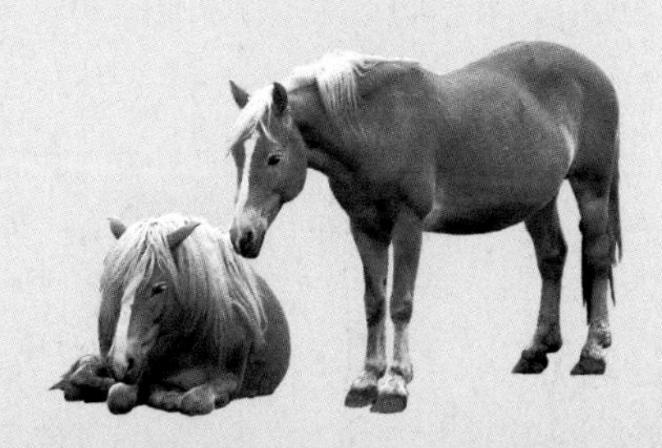

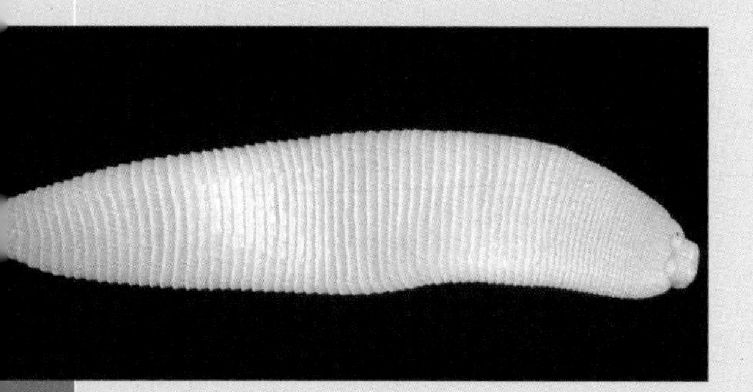

A tapeworm, fortunately rarely found.
Photo: Pfitzer

A collection of bot larvae on the stomach lining.
Photo: Pfitzer

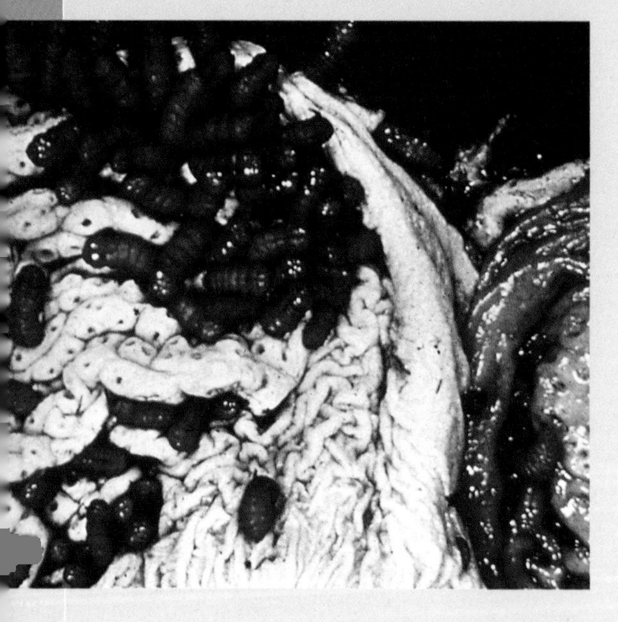

penetrate the tendons, tendon sheaths, the nuchal ligament and the fluids of the eyes.

Tapeworms (Anaplocephala perfoliata)

This worm can reach up to 80 cm in length, and for its three to five month life cycle uses a moss mite as an intermediate host. The larvae, together with the moss mite, survive in the bedding or the paddock and are ingested by the horse. Tapeworms are very difficult to spot and are not easily identified using the routine worming tests. Tests on droppings may show no sign of tapeworms, even when horses are infested.

Liver fluke (Fasciola hepatica)

Fortunately, the liver fluke is not often found. Its main host is cattle. They are often found in mild and humid climates, such as in Ireland. The four-month life cycle of this worm requires a small snail as the intermediate host, and where there are no snails the liver fluke cannot survive. Infestation causes anaemia and weight loss. Routine worming does not control the liver fluke.

Bots (Gastrophilus)

It is worth noting that this is not a worm, but an insect. The maggot-like larvae of the bot fly pose a significant risk. New research has shown that infestation by bot flies is increasing. Every second horse is affected, and horses play host to bots throughout the year. The worst time for attacks is from December until March, so treatment should be given starting at the end of November and continuing until mid December, and subsequently repeated. Infestation leads to anaemia, colic and loss of performance. The bot fly sheds yellow eggs from July until September, onto the legs of horses. The horses scratch and lick, thereby ingesting the eggs, which develop into larvae in the stomach. You can reduce the burden of parasites by removing the eggs from the horses' legs in late summer.

How can such small organisms harm such large animals?

The fact is, worms are extremely numerous. They cause serious damage to the intestines due to the migration of the larvae, and are implicated in the following symptoms:

- loss of performance
- loss of condition
- loss of appetite
- dull coat
- itchy tail
- anaemia
- swollen legs (or sheath area)
- circulatory problems
- liver damage
- breathing difficulties
- diarrhoea
- colic

Some of these symptoms can have deadly consequences, especially diarrhoea and colic.

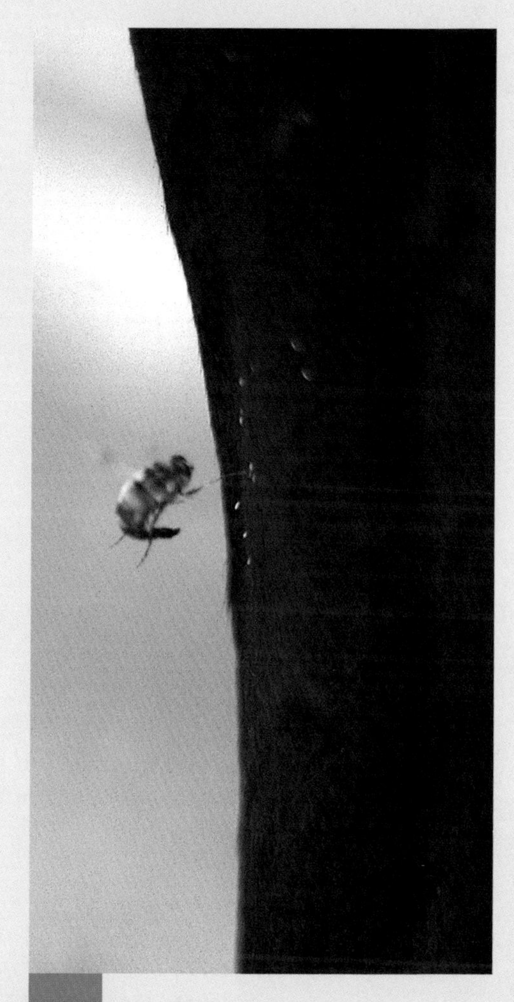

The perfect spot for a bot fly's eggs.
Photo: H. Ende

The telltale signs of bot flies. The eggs stick to the horse's skin and should be removed.
Photo: H. Ende

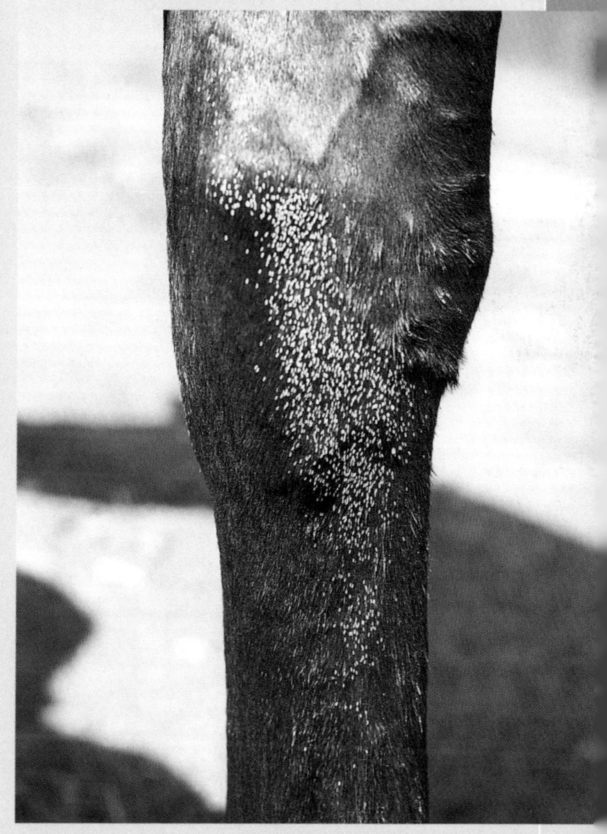

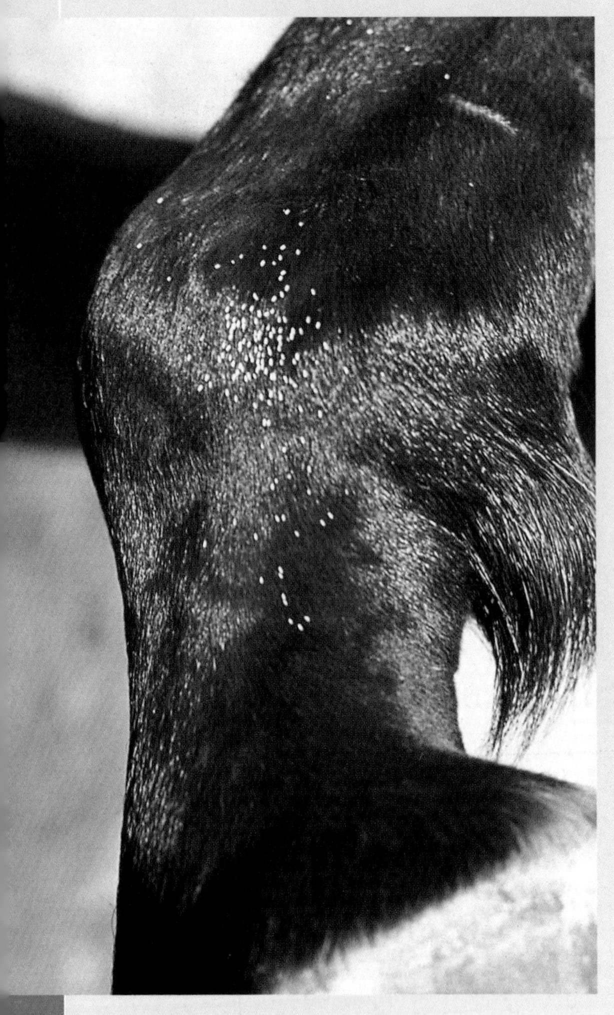

Examine your horse thoroughly, from top to bottom.
Photo: H. Ende

It is generally the case that some horses are more susceptible to illness than others. Added to that is the possibility of genetic susceptibility to parasite infestation. And horses which are lower in the pecking order have to graze where stronger horses choose not to. This way, weaker horses are forced to graze on rougher patches where more parasites tend to live. When a single horse in a herd shows signs of illness or loss of performance, it could well be a worm-related problem. When in doubt, discuss the problem with your vet, and review your hygiene measures, pasture management and worming strategy. Have droppings and blood tested, and the affected horse or horses examined.

Normally a parasite does not kill its host – after all, it needs the host to live off. The ideal situation, from the parasite's point of view, is where it can take what it needs from the host on a regular basis without causing any serious damage. Parasites survive as species by multiplying quickly, developing resistance to medication, being untreatable during migration of the larvae, and by having resistant eggs.

Knowledge of their life cycles is important, because this is the only way we can successfully plan our defence. In the case of roundworms, for instance, which have no intermediate host, every stage of the life cycle occurs in the horse, as eggs, larvae and then adult worms. Their progress must be interrupted during as many stages as possible. With parasites which spend part of their life cycles away from the horse, there is the added possibility of removing the intermediate host in order to fight the infestation more successfully.

Horses host different stages of the developing worms, which means that there are likely to be various species of worms living in the horse at all times.

It is important in the battle against worms to keep in mind that at certain stages of their life cycles they are beyond the reach of medication, and that not all worms can be treated with the same active ingredients. In tests of their droppings you will generally find various eggs, because horses almost always have a variety of worms.

While a completely parasite-free horse may be a near impossibility, we can at least reduce the burden for our horses by taking proper hygiene measures and administering appropriate prophylactic and therapeutic worming treatment.

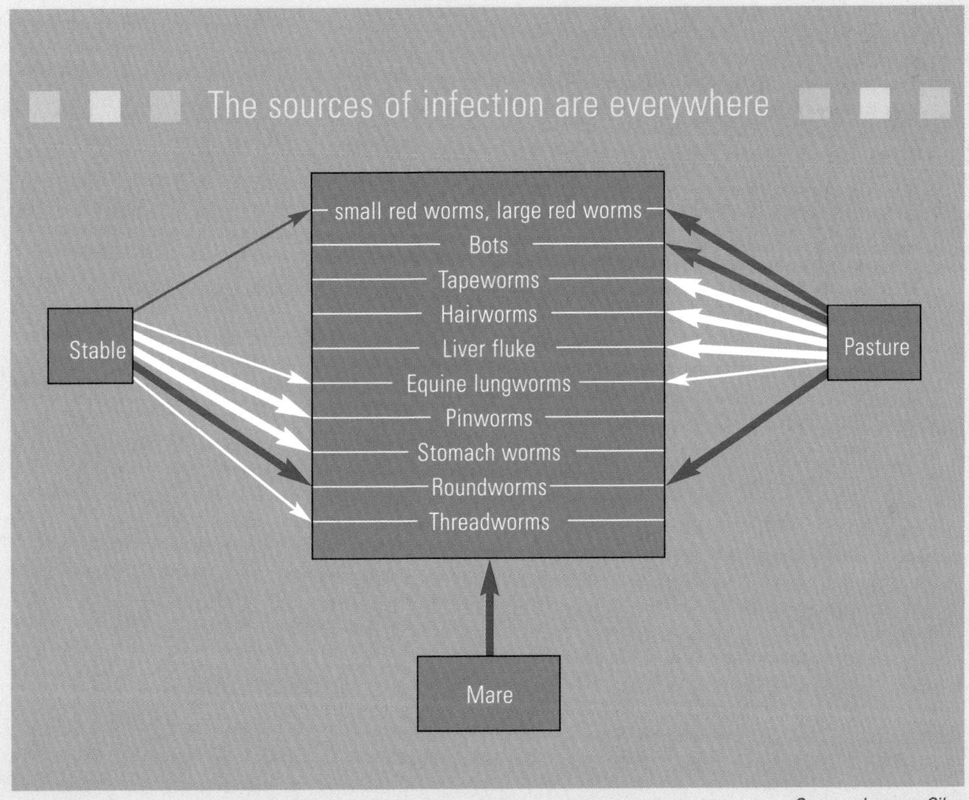

Source: Janssen-Cilag

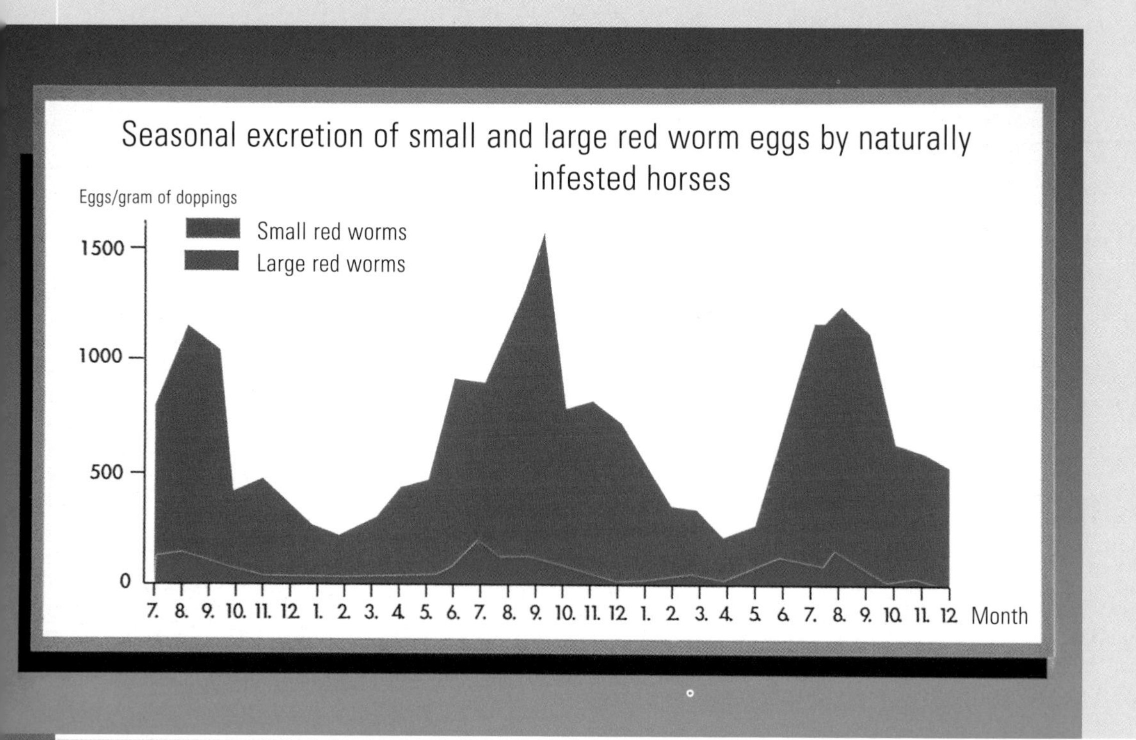

Source: Pfitzner GmbH

Tip

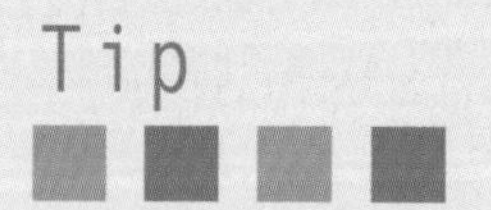

There are no shortcuts to pasture hygiene!

Principles of hygiene

The priority here must be careful maintenance of the yard and pasture.

Stable management
Daily mucking out and regular cleaning of stables is to be highly recommended. In ideal conditions, the walls of stables are smooth and dry, to prevent larvae sticking to them.

Horses should not be fed from the floor, in order to minimise contamination. While the use of a hayrack decreases the risk of parasite infestation, this can contribute to postural problems (backache) and can also be a burden to the horse's airways.

Pasture management

Good management is in the interest of all horses that are put out to pasture, even those which go out for only a few hours each day.

It is extremely important to allow pastures a rest period, even in a small stable yard. It is preferable to rest a pasture for at least four months during the year, but if that is impossible, even six weeks' rest will make a dramatic impact on the parasite load.

The ideal situation would be to alternate pastures on a yearly basis with sheep and

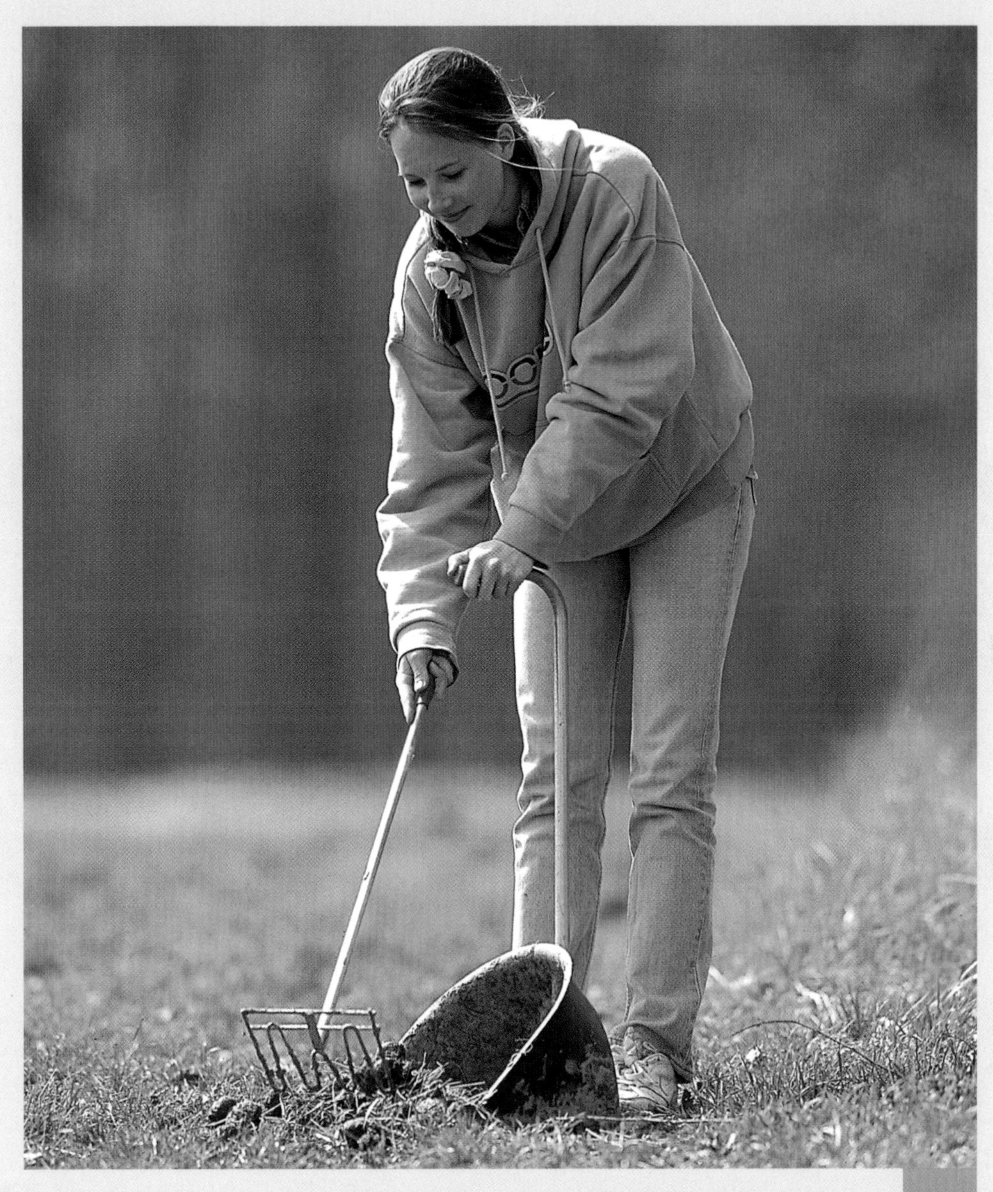

Only when you pick up droppings on a regular basis (at least every three days) will it be effective in the control of parasites. Photo: S. Stuewer

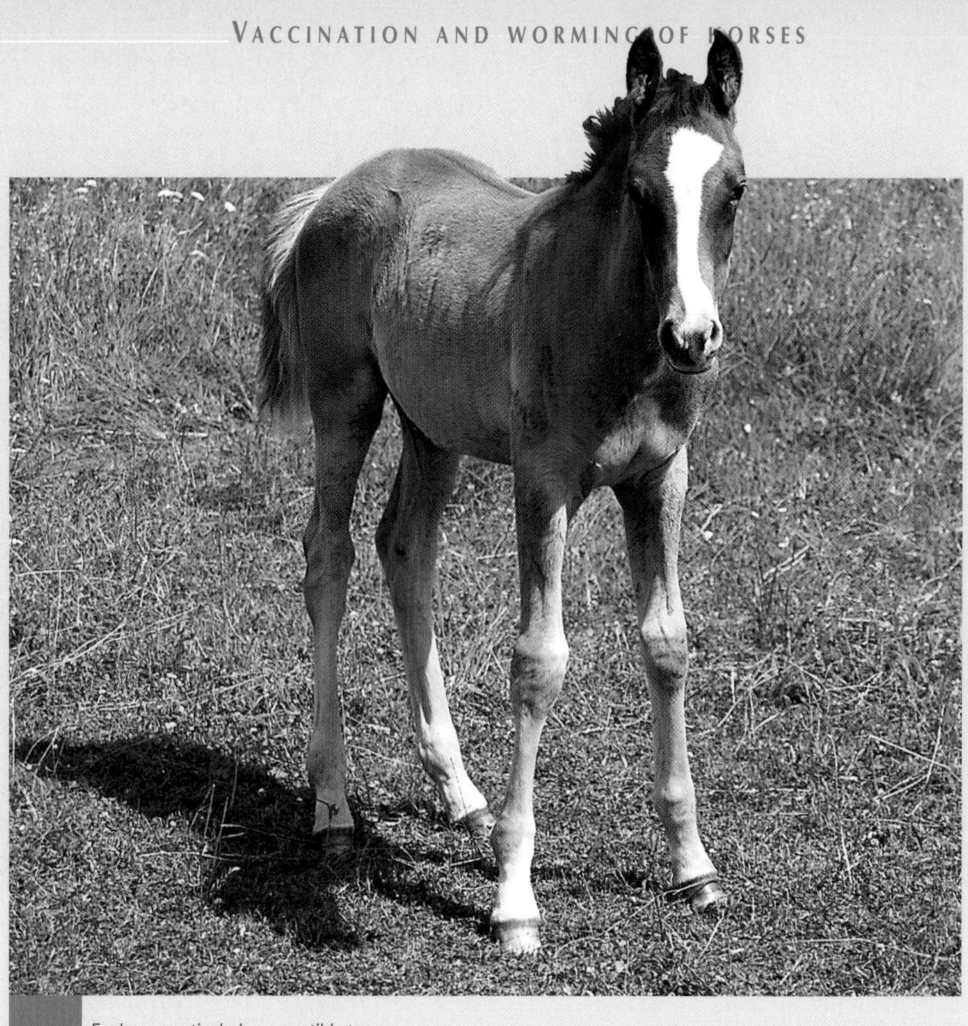

Foals are particularly susceptible to parasite infestations. Photo: R. Ettl

cattle. These animals can ingest horses' parasites without harm, just as parasites from cattle can do no harm to horses.

It is helpful, before you allow horses onto a pasture, to mow the grass and cordon off a small area. By moving the fence daily, you can regulate the grazing of the pasture and control over-eating.

Over-grazing should be avoided – ideally there should be no more than two horses per hectare of pasture. Pasture should be well drained and reasonably dry.

It takes only three days from the moment a horse leaves droppings until the migration of the larvae begins. This is the time within which you should remove the droppings. Only regular removal of droppings is of any benefit. In this way, the parasite load can be dramatically reduced. It takes only a few weeks to contaminate a pasture, but it can take years to get it disinfected. Acquire a droppings scoop and rake, and a well-suspended light barrow, because this is a task which is easier with the right tools. Draw up a rota which shows whose turn it is to remove the droppings. Members of golf clubs pay a lot of money to walk across grass with carts and tools in search of small balls.... By removing droppings you promote your own health (regular exercise in fresh air), have time to let your thoughts wander, and at the same time do something which contributes to your horses' well-being. It is not that much work either – seven horses produce about two barrowfuls of droppings a day, which should take less than 30 minutes to collect.

An easier but less effective method is to rake apart the droppings to let the sun dry out the eggs. Unfortunately, nobody can rake so thoroughly that every single egg is exposed, and in any case, British summers are seldom hot enough to kill the eggs. And mind that you do not simply rake the parasite eggs all over the pasture, so that even the cleverest horses cannot graze around them!

Horses which have just been wormed will immediately pick up new larvae if they are turned out in a contaminated pasture, and the whole exercise will have been futile. It therefore makes sense, as is common practice, to worm horses three days before swapping pastures. Better still, worm the horses, then put them in the new pasture and collect the droppings on a daily basis for three days. To stable horses after worming, if they are normally turned out, is asking for trouble. The treatment of the parasites is already a burden to the horse, and the conversion from grass to hay, plus the stress of unfamiliar confinement, is a recipe for colic. Yearlings and foals should not be turned out on the same pasture for two years in a row. Foals are particularly susceptible to parasitic infestation. In ideal circumstances, foals should be turned out in pastures which have been used by cattle and then rested the previous year. Foals that are reared on pasture often survive a mild infestation of roundworms and go on to develop a good defence mechanism. Foals which are born early in the season, and are kept indoors for a few months, are not exposed to this mild infestation and can fall gravely ill when turned out into mildly contaminated pastures.

Proper pasture management minimises the risk of infestation, and regular worm treatment can reduce it even further. With good pasture management, the interval between worming treatments can be extended to the maximum.

An extremely contaminated pasture can be prepared for horses by ploughing it. Time must then be allowed for the new grass to grow, and in an ideal world it should also be mown at least once.

New horses that are being introduced to a group should be presumed to be infested, and should be wormed as soon as they come to the yard. Repeat the treatment at the recommended time, and only then introduce the new horse to the herd. From then on it should be included in the existing worming plan.

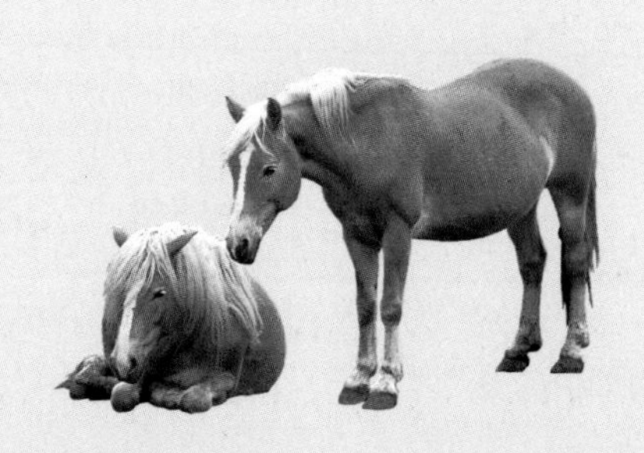

Prophylactic treatment of worms

In principle, all adult horses should be wormed at least four times a year, all at the same time and using the same drug.

The drugs available differ in their recommended intervals between use. The recommendation might be, for example, to repeat treatment after two to three months. This means worming horses in frequently changing herds every two months, and every three months for horses kept in stables or in isolated herds on well-kept pastures.

In individual cases, horses which are always kept in isolated paddocks can be wormed selectively. To minimise any risk, it is wise to perform an egg count on a sample of droppings from each horse. When more than 200 red worm eggs are found per gram of droppings, then worming is due.

Tip

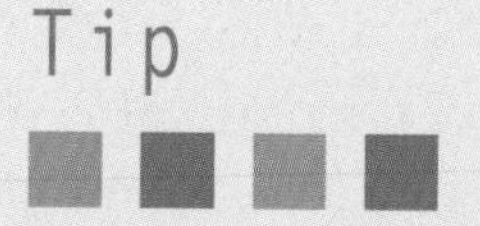

Worm all horses with medication containing the same active ingredient.

An indication of parasite infestation can also be gained by means of a blood test. The proportion of a type of white blood cell, the eosinophil leukocytes, is increased in the differential blood profile of affected animals. Foals and yearlings must be wormed more frequently.

New additions to the herd must always first be isolated and wormed before being permitted to join the other horses.

In the first three months of pregnancy, mares should not be subjected to any medication, including worming. Discuss a plan of action

Strategic worming plan

(This is only an example, which can be adapted to suit individual requirements. Worming four times a year is the minimum recommendation.)

	First Year	Second Year	Third Year
March	Benzimidazole	Pyrantel	Avermectin
June	Benzimidazole	Pyrantel	Avermectin
September:	Benzimidazole	Pyrantel	Avermectin
December:	Avermectin	Avermectin	Avermectin

for the rest of the pregnancy with your vet. It is advisable to give the mare ivermectin on the day she foals, to prevent the excretion of large numbers of threadworms in her milk.

To avoid the problem of resistance, the active ingredient should be rotated on a yearly basis. Please note, it is the active in-gredient, not the brand, that is rotated on a yearly basis, and not every time. Unfortunately, many horse owners just buy a different-looking packet. In most cases this is insufficient. There are three groups of active ingredients and should be alternated annually. To rotate to another wormer containing an active ingredient from the same group does nothing to improve worm control. An egg count on a sample of droppings can assess the extent of worm infestation, and can be used to test the effectiveness of the worming plan.

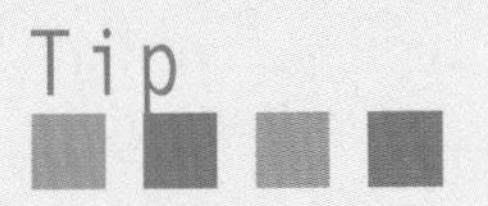

Avermectin is the only active ingredient that works against bots.

Avermectins

Ivermectin belongs to this group, and is available on the market as Eqvalan and Furexel. These are essentially the same paste from two different manufacturers, the variation being in the packaging and price. The second active substance in this group is moxidectin, which is available as Equest.

These substances function by interrupting the transmission of nerve impulses in the worm. This leads to paralysis and death of the worm.

Here are two different packets, each containing the same active ingredients group: Avermectin. Eqvalan contains ivermectin, moxidectin is available in Equest. Photo: HJS

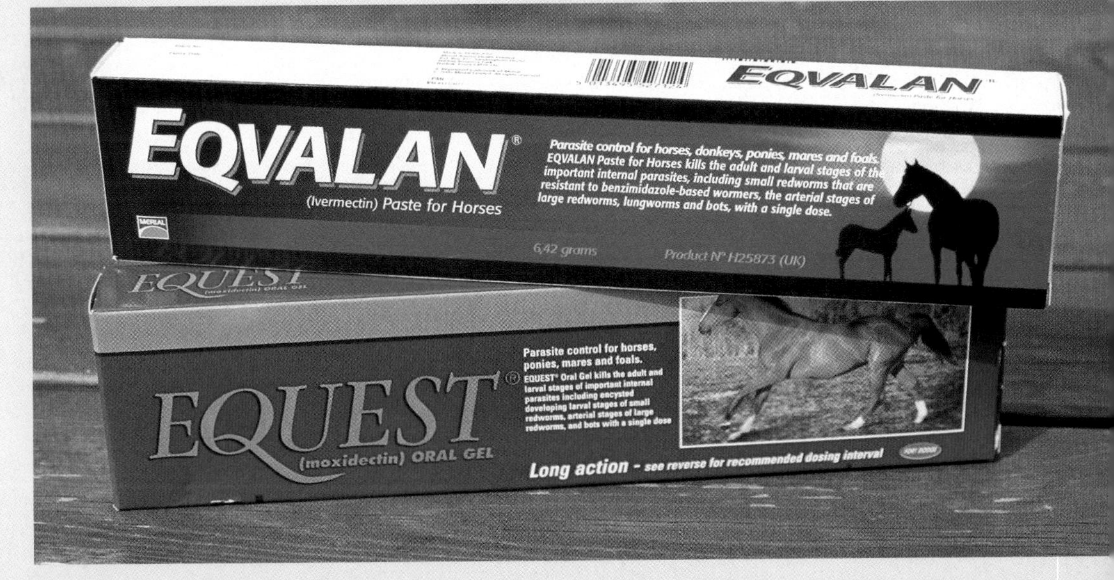

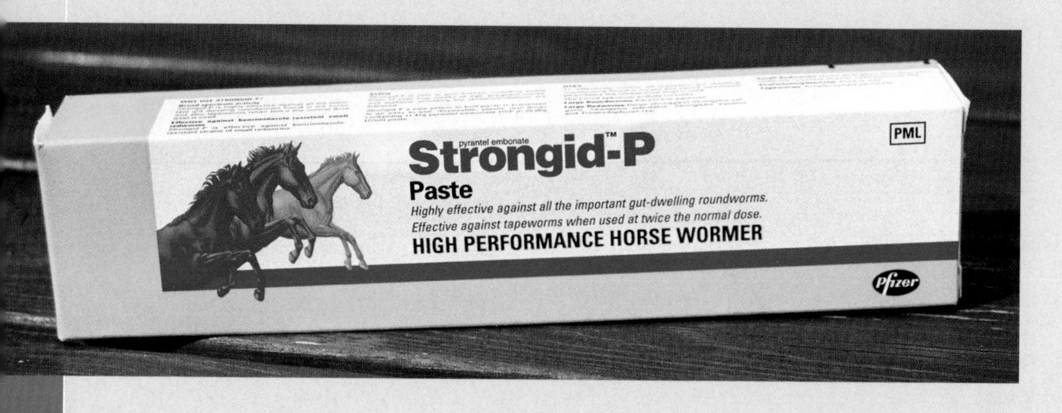

This drug contains pyrantel as the active ingredient. Using a double dose it also acts against tapeworms. Photo: HJS

In the standard dosage, these substances destroy red worms, pinworms, roundworms, lungworms, threadworms, stomach worms, filarial nematodes and bots. Moxidectin is the only active ingredient which can destroy the larvae of the small red worm while they are in the wall of the intestines.

When a horse suffers with microfilariae, this can lead to swelling and itchiness. If it does not improve within a day, a veterinarian must be consulted.

Pyrimidins

Pyrantel embonate (also called pyrantel pamoate) belongs to this group, and is available as Strongid or Pyratape on the market.

Pyrantel works in the intestines only, by paralysing the worms. This means it is only effective against adult worms and, to a lesser extent, the eggs.

Pyrantel destroys large and small red worms, pinworms, and roundworms.

At higher doses, pyrantel is used to treat tapeworms.

Caution:

Severely weakened foals, infested by roundworms, can suffer blockage of the intestines as a result.

Caution:

When large numbers of larvae are present, there may be side effects when the worms die en masse.

Benzimidazoles

All other worming products belong to this group. The various active ingredients they contain are diverse in their functions, which is important in therapeutic treatment. In prophylactic use, alternating between these drugs is not very useful, as some worms can develop a resistance to drugs in the benzimidazole group. The active ingredient fenbendazole is available in paste, liquid and granules as Panacur, and also in granule form as Zerofen. It works by disturbing the worms' intake of nourishment so they then starve.

In the standard dosage, these substances destroy large adult red worms, small adult red worms that are not resistant to benzimidazole, pinworms and roundworms.

Used five days in a row, fenbendazole destroys threadworms, immature small red worms and, to some extent, the larvae of small red worm.

Panacur paste is now available on the market which has a better taste, boasting apple and cinnamon flavour!

The active ingredient mebendazole has a similar effect, and is available as Telmin. It treats the same spectrum of parasites using a standard dose, and also destroys lungworms.

Prophylactic treatment

- at least four times a year
- all horses in the same herd at the same time
- at the same time as pasture changes, with daily removal of droppings for the first three days after treatment
- alternate active ingredients annually
- treatment against bots in December for horses at pasture
- regular egg counts from droppings to test effectiveness

Very old horses, or those which display symptoms of worm-related damage, can undergo a five-day therapeutic treatment with fenbendazole in February.

Foals should be wormed from their third to sixth week onwards. They should be wormed together with the mare, and the worming must be repeated every eight weeks. From six months of age, the foals (and their mothers) can be included in the normal worming plan. On the day of foaling, the mare should be given ivermectin to counteract the excretion of threadworms in the milk, and in this way protect the foal. This is also important if mares are to be covered again the next time they come into season. It is better to abstain from giving any medication during the first three months of pregnancy.

Therapeutic treatment of worms

If an egg count is done on a sample of droppings which reveals a specific worm infestation, treatment beyond that specified by the worming plan may be required. Taking a new egg count a short time later will test the effectiveness of the worming treatment. The egg count should be reduced by at least 70 per cent. The rest of the herd should also be observed.

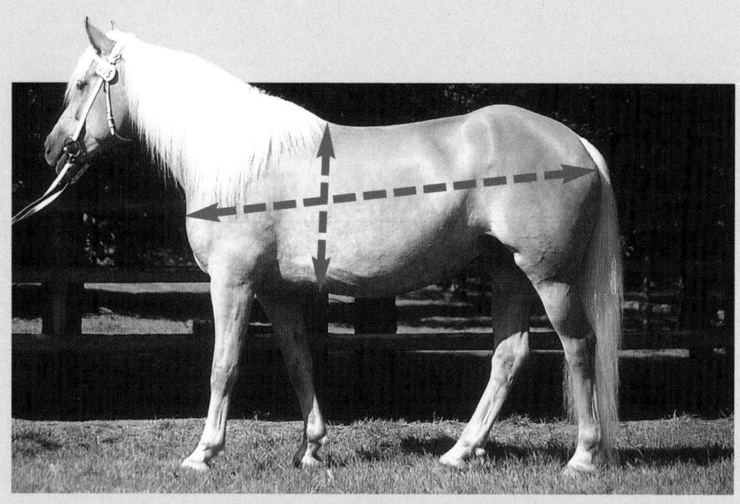

You can determine the weight of your horse by measuring the circumference of the girth and the length of the body. Photo: A. Schmelzer

$$\text{Weight (kg)} = \frac{\text{girth (cm)} \times \text{girth (cm)} \times \text{length of body (cm)}}{11900}$$

How to worm a horse

The amount of drug which should be administered depends on the horse's bodyweight. If you do not know the bodyweight of your horse, you can go to the nearest livestock scale or lorry weighbridge. You can also use the above formula to calculate it.

The paste comes in syringe form, containing enough for a 600 kg horse. With most pastes, one can adjust the amount given by turning a little wheel to provide the correct dose for a smaller horse. There is generally no need to panic if the whole dose is accidentally administered, as with most wormers a double dose is not harmful.

The most important factor is to avoid giving too little. On the one hand, it will not be as effective, and on the other, it can allow the worms to develop a resistance. To ensure that the right amount is given to a difficult horse, it is always better to have a spare dose to hand. This avoids you having to go and buy another dose after the stable walls, your clothes, and the horse's nose are covered with paste. When you have already lost control, it is it is much more likely that things will go wrong all over again.

The surest way to administer the drug is in paste form. As a paste, or the granular variety, it can be mixed into the horse's feed, but do ensure that everything is eaten in one session. The wormer can be bought from your vet, who will give you any necessary advice. It can also be bought from a veterinary pharmacy, or some feed stores, with a prescription.

How to administer paste:

- If you are inexperienced in giving treatments, breathe deeply and relax; ideally have a helper.
- Wear safe shoes and a hard hat, to prevent possible injury.
- Conceal the syringe, ready to be used, in a pocket.
- Use a head collar and lead rope.
- Make sure the horse's mouth is empty – a mouthful of feed or hay makes it easy for the animal to spit the paste out.
- Move calmly and confidently.
- Stand on the left of your horse, put your left hand on its nose and take the syringe in your other hand without the horse noticing.
- Put the syringe in the side of the mouth, at an angle.
- Squeeze the paste promptly onto the horse's tongue.
- Twist the syringe when you remove it, to smear any remaining paste on the tongue.
- Reward your horse when the paste has been swallowed.

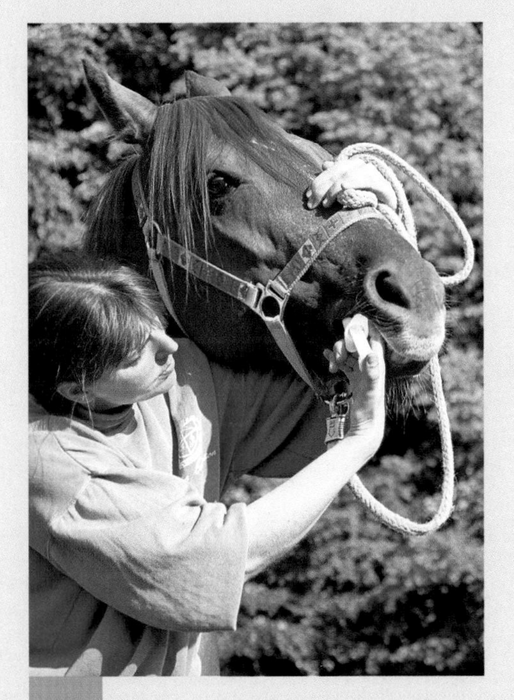

The right way. Photo: HJS

Do not be tempted to buy any wormer on the basis of its cheapness. The risk to the horse and the expense of any extra treatment needed if it does not work are unpleasant and avoidable. After all, you would not buy sweets to cure a headache, just because they are colourful, cheap and widely available.

Prevention is better than cure!

Imprint

Translated by: Desiree Gerber
Edited by: Andrea Chee
Design and composition: Ravenstein Brain Pool
Photographs: A. Schmelzer, S. Stuewer
Printed by Westermann Druck, Zwickau

Printed in Germany.
ISBN 3-86127-931-2

Other Cadmos Books

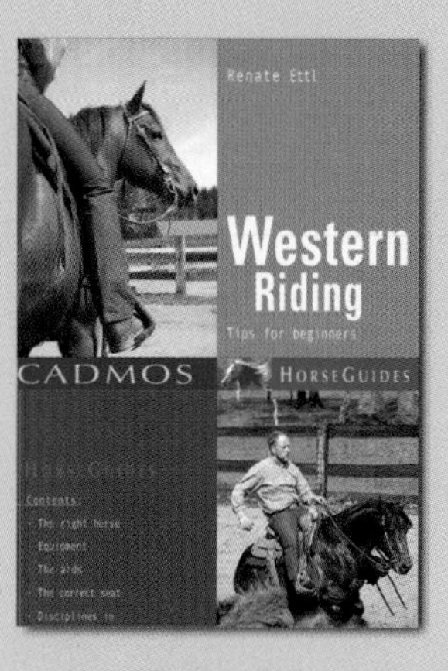

Renate Ettl

Western Riding

A perfect guide for beginners and those who wish to change to Western Riding.

Paperback, 32 colour pages
ISBN 3-86127-933-9

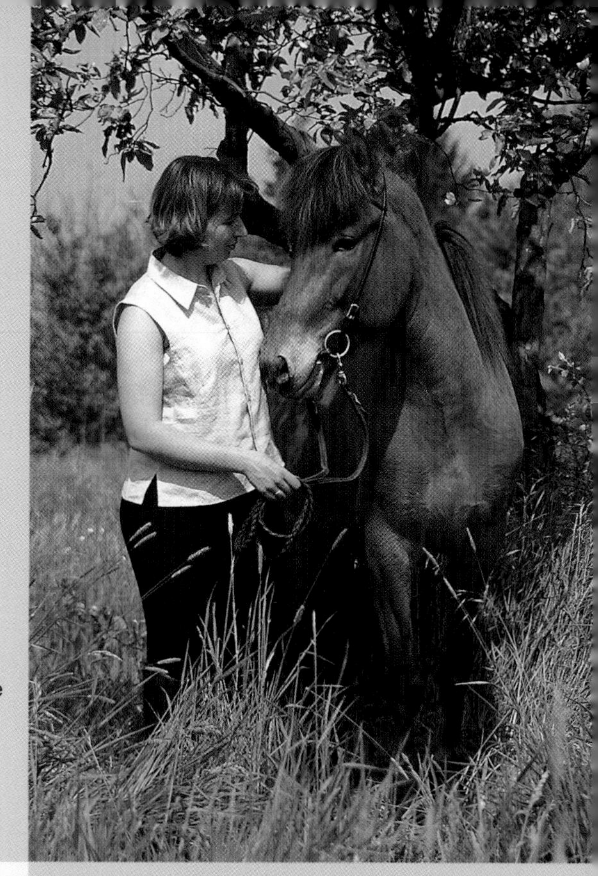

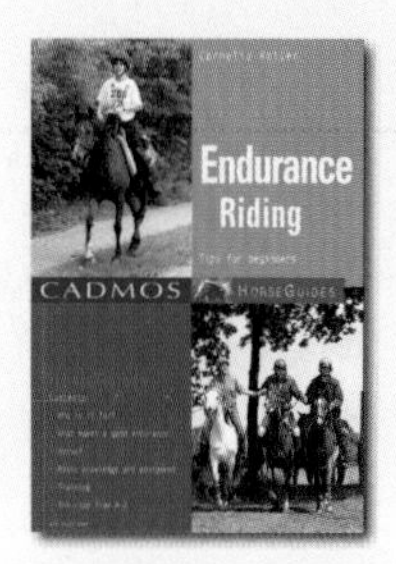

Cornelia Koller

Endurance Riding

This horse guide contains a wealth of basic knowledge for all beginners, wanting to know more about this fascinating sport.

Paperback, 32 colour pages
ISBN 3-86127-930-4

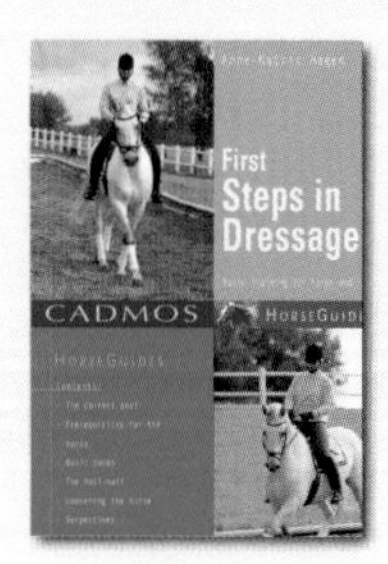

Anne-Katrin Hagen

First Steps in Dressage

The author describes lessons in serpentines, half-halt, basic paces with lengthening and leg-yielding.

Paperback, 32 colour pages
ISBN 3-86127-932-0

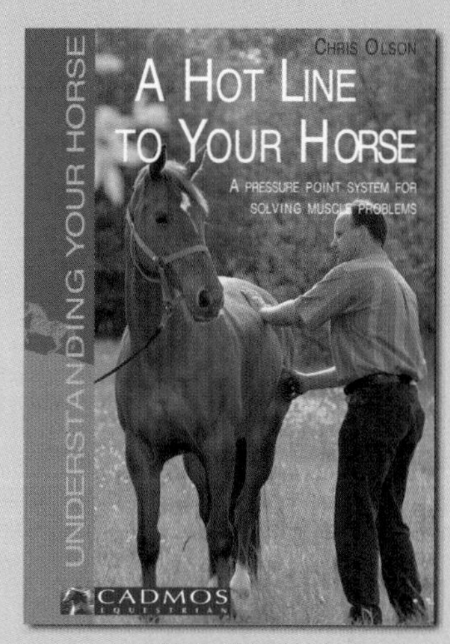

Chris Olson

A Hot Line to Your Horse

A Hot Line to Your Horse sets out an effective, easily comprehensible method which you can quickly master and use to enhance your horse´s well-being and willingness to perform.

Paperback, 80 colour pages
ISBN 3-86127-901-0

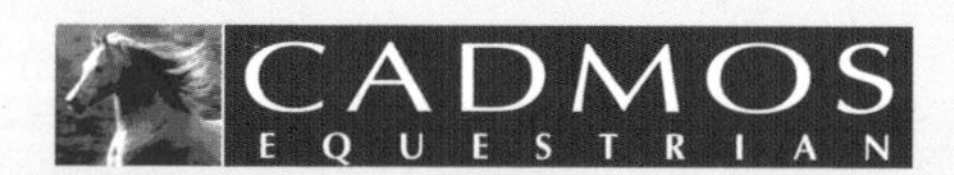

For further information: Cadmos Equestrian
The Editmaster Company
28 Langham Place Northampton NN2 6
Tel. 01604 715915 Fax: 06104 791209